Outsic Hearts

HEROIC STORIES FROM THE LEPROSY HOSPITAL IN MYANMAR

✻

Gary Watkins

T4T Press

Nashville, Tennessee

Love for Myanmar

305 Ten Oaks Drive

Georgetown, Texas 78633

www.LoveforMyanmar.org

Book Layout ©2017 BookDesignTemplates.com

Ordering Information:

Quantity sales. Special discounts are available on quantity purchases by corporations, associations, and others. For details, contact the "Special Sales Department" at the address above.

Outside Our Hearts/Gary Watkins. —1st ed.

ISBN 978-1-9808886-2-8

Contents

FORWARD 2

GOD'S CALL 4

MY EPIPHANY 6

ABOUT MYANMAR 9

LEPROSY MINISTRY 12

HOSPITAL GROUNDS 14

LEPROSY DISEASE 19

HOSPITAL STAFF 21

LEPROSY VILLAGE 27

FIRST IMPRESSIONS 29

LEPROSY PATIENTS 33

RELIGIOUS PERSPECTIVES 45

PERSONAL REFLECTIONS 50

MY PLEA (TO GOD) 60

MY PLEA (TO YOU) 62

WHEN (A PRAYER FOR YOU) 69

JOIN US 71

To the staff, patients, and families of the Mawlamyine Christian Leprosy Hospital for battling together against the disease of isolation

Don't be afraid to speak from personal experience; in many ways, those vulnerable moments will be the key that unlocks a hardened heart.
–LUIS PALAU

IN APPRECIATION

TO THE LEPROSY hospital staff for the deep honor by which you serve your patients, the deep preoccupation you have with protecting their dignity, and the deep resolve you have for sharing God's love in one of the darkest corners of this life.

To Stuart Briscoe, Jim Denison, Tony Evans, Greg Laurie, John Piper, Charles Stanley, Rick Warren, and James Emery White for your unswerving determination, firm moral convictions, and unchanging concern to help us know God better. Thank you for your writings which provided me with the spiritual insights that helped me more fully understand the importance of a "fighting faith."

To my wife for her keen editorial skills, gift of direction, and loving frankness which collectively gave a recognizable purpose to my otherwise scattered observations.

To Dan Lancaster for his administrative insight, calming presence, and affirming mind-set, which reduced the chaos normally accompanying the torturous publication process.

Most especially, to my God to whom alone be the glory:

Not to us, Lord, not to us, but to your name give glory because of Your faithful love and Your truth. Psalm 115:1 (NIV)

FORWARD

... for man looks on the outward appearance, but the Lord looks at the heart.1Samuel 16:7 (NIV)

AS CHRISTIANS, how can we believe and say that "He lives within my heart" when we exclude "the least of these" from our love? There is an unfortunate distance between God's love for us and our love for others. Just because we claim to have God's love within us, doesn't make it so. It seems reasonable that Christians should consider themselves obligated to examine their hearts continually, to ensure they connect faithfully to the unconditional love central to the Christian message.

People's lives, the lives of lepers in Myanmar specifically, have shown that they placed their trust in religious beliefs which have provided empty answers. In Myanmar, there is an opportunity for Christianity to rekindle these lives and guide them toward everlasting hope. Right now, these people are outside our hearts while they wrestle with a religious upbringing fundamentally contrary to Christianity. Nonetheless, we believe this is the ministry in which Jesus Christ would involve Himself.

The key is you; however, thus far, few are receptive to the idea of traveling to the other side of the world to endure the inconveniences commonplace in a developing country. Most are hiding from this Christian responsibility, preferring to manipulate the principle of "serving others" to suit their own spiritual fulfillment. Some are intimidated by the distance and the annoying logistics of security screenings, layovers and rushed transfers in strange airports, and long stints in cramped airline seats. Others are intimidated by the cultural differences—different languages, different customs, different food, different money, different people, different landscape, different laws.

One truth, I think, is that we are intimidated by failure. In our attempts to avoid failure, we construct situations to minimize our risks rather than dare to rely on God's strengths. We want success on our terms. We want there to be witnesses to our good deeds. We want the limelight. We want our family and friends to think glowingly of us.

Another truth, I think, is that to be unnoticed personally is to place the halo where it properly belongs...with God. Because we believe this ministry began from God's heart, we believe for those who willingly follow, their service will become a joy not a sacrifice.

In the meantime, until we adjust our focus of Christian service to reflect that He is truly within us, others, such as the lepers in Myanmar, will remain outside our hearts.

CHAPTER 1

※

GOD'S CALL

A man's heart plans his way, but the Lord directs his steps.
Proverbs 16:9 (NIV)

FLYING AT 32,000 FEET and traveling at 565 mph over the Pacific Ocean is not a fitting time to change your mind about a trip. I sat uneasy in my seat, questioning my decision to travel to a country about which I knew very little. Compounding my difficulty was realizing what little I had to offer the mission team.

Although a Christian, I was not a regular student of the Bible. In fact, as best I can recall, I had not been to church for 10 years. The details of my absence are not important. It is enough to state that, despite my genuine anger toward God for how my life was progressing, there were no good reasons for such a lengthy separation.

There I was starting my journey, and I was searching for the emergency exit to put a merciful end to my anguish over allowing my emotional reaction to a mission trip presentation at church lead me 10,000 miles away, to Myanmar. I had no talents and had never been on a mission trip. Of what possible value could I be to this team and their cause?

What unfolded over the next 15 days changed my life. I had seen many of the same images of orphaned children you may have seen on television or when leafing through articles with pictures of desperate faces. On that trip, at age 58, I learned the difference between physical poverty and spiritual starvation.

Despite the overwhelming oppression surrounding every facet of their daily lives, I learned much from the people of Myanmar. I learned what it means to share when you have so little. I learned what it means to be faithful when surrounded by evil. I learned what it means to love when there is so much sorrow.

I have just returned from my fifteenth trip to Myanmar. Between trips, I have co-founded a nonprofit called *Love for Myanmar*, a Christian-based organization offering various programs to strengthen families within and from Myanmar.

In Myanmar, we are involved with ministering to hundreds of abandoned and orphaned children, developing neighborhood schools, and establishing a network of house churches, and more. In Austin, Texas, we are involved in aiding Myanmar refugees immigrating from refugee camps in Thailand.

As I reflected on my first trip, I decided that despite the thousands of miles covered, the longest part of my journey was traveling the distance between my mind and my heart. It was that rainy Sunday morning, in July 2007, when I discovered God's plan for me.

CHAPTER 2

MY EPIPHANY

How many people have you made homesick for God? --
OSWALD CHAMBERS

HEAVEN NUDGED its clouds and the rain kept coming. There were no drops, just layers of water stretching upwards as far as I could see. It was Sunday, and we were in a distant land, in an impoverished area of the former Mon state capital, preparing to visit a small church. As we neared the church, the rain intensified and the narrow, dirt road quickly became a quagmire disappearing in to the surrounding landscape.

We finally made it to the church where the pastor greeted us, and we visited for a while. As we emerged from our discussion, we walked toward an opening in the bamboo structure and, through the sheets of rain still pummeling the countryside, we could hear the voices of the congregation as they approached their church. The pastor led us to the area where the service was to be held, and following his lead, we sat in the front row.

The service began a short while later and unfolded warmly from song to song, with an occasional comment or prayer from the pastor or church leader. Then the pastor told the congregation that they had special guests among them and each would share encouraging words with them. The previous day, the pastor asked if one of us could provide the sermon.

Fortunately, we had someone in our group of four who had such experience, and he agreed to give the sermon. Now, we all were expected to talk to the congregation. My greatest fear was gripping my entire body and squeezing my mind to the point that I was now totally void of any thoughts, anything meaningful to share. I was the last to speak.

As I rose from my chair and walked the few steps to the front, I just knew everyone would begin to wonder about that sound and would soon realize it was my heart beating, trying to escape my chest, trying to hide in some corner of the room until this moment passed. But at that moment, there was something you could no longer hear...the rain.

When I turned to face the congregation, none of whom I had seen because we were in the front row with our backs to them, my senses were flooded with a peace I have never experienced. The sun's rays began to wander into the room; a fresh, crisp air began to drift over the gathering; and then, I became mesmerized by the expressions on the people's faces. Each person was glimmering while blending into a collective radiance that filled my eyes with joy. I have never felt more connected to a moment, closer to God.

To this day, I have no recollection of what I shared with that congregation, and I haven't asked my traveling companions either, being afraid of what I would learn. I have no recollection of my comments because I truly believe God made me deaf to my own words. God wanted my attention to be on what He was saying to me:

Here, in front of you, are 100 persecuted persons, many who have lost family members, many who have been tortured themselves, many who have had their land taken, and many who have had their dignity as human beings ripped from their souls. But, their faith is their connection to one another, their bond to hope, and their promise to me to forgive and live the Christian life, no matter the personal cost. How far will your faith take you?

I had come 10,000 miles to Myanmar to discover I hadn't yet taken a step. God carried me to this place and positioned me for the real journey—the journey of faith. It was time for me to take my first step—the only step God cannot take for you. That step of faith which, once taken, illuminates your purpose. For me, it is my desire to use my love and respect for the people of Myanmar to bring about positive change in their lives.

CHAPTER 3

LOVE FOR MYANMAR

I refuse to see any problem as anything less than an opportunity to see God. -- *MAX LUCADO*

MYANMAR IS A COUNTRY in Southeast Asia bordered by China, Thailand, Bangladesh, and India. The country boasts a large coastline, stunning mountainous regions, and everything between. Its three largest cities are Yangon, Mandalay, and the capital, Naypyidaw. It is a mainly Buddhist country.

In 1962, a military junta took over Myanmar. Under this regime, Myanmar was subject to some of the world's most terrible human rights violations while suffering from extreme poverty and malnutrition. The country has recently been moving toward a more democratic process.

After five decades of military rule, Nobel Peace Laureate Aung San Suu Kyi's party won a landslide victory on November 8, 2015. Although the military continues to wield substantial power, many in Myanmar and throughout the world are hopeful there will be a peaceful transition to democracy.

Myanmar is amid hugely challenging transitions: from conflict to peace, from authoritarian to democratic rule, and from a closed to an open economy. Myanmar is a small stage on this earth, and its people with leprosy equally insignificant...forgotten. We need to think about surrendering our plans, so God can carry out His. However, few of us are humble enough to accept the gift of sacrifice and surrender our self-concerns to intercede for the lives of strangers.

Regardless of Myanmar's many challenges, *Love for Myanmar* intends to continue its ministries. We don't see politicians. We don't see military personnel. We don't see Buddhists. We see people—honorable, humble, and hurting. We intend to continue listening to their perspectives, focusing on their needs, and addressing their hurts.

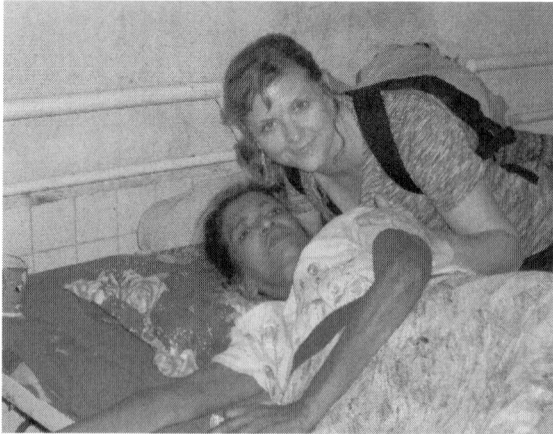

Myanmar is a land afraid of religious questions, which has resulted in a people spiritually retreating from most of the world. There are few opportunities to exercise your religious curiosity, to search for the reasons to help you make sense of the world in which you find yourself, to struggle and doubt about those ideas which have been no small part of your upbringing. How can they know their religion is telling them the truth? There must be a way to build a bridge between their unexamined ideas of Buddhism and Christianity.

This is an invitation to Christians to experience God working through them to touch others for Christ. These lepers and their families need to know the Lord you fell in love with.

No matter how you have meandered spiritually, the twists of your journey of faith, the distractions of earthly blessings, don't undervalue the enjoyment God has wrapped around the challenges He has placed in your path.

Before your time on this earth dissolves, dare to serve others as if this life is not the only world that matters.

If Jesus returned today, where would He find you; what would you be doing?

CHAPTER 4

LEPROSY MINISTRY

God measures success by obedience. -- *DR. JIM DENISON*

DURING A TRIP TO MYANMAR in the Spring of 2014, *Love for Myanmar*'s founders and their spouses were led to the Leprosy Hospital in Mawlamyine located in the Mon state. What was observed stirred a mixture of emotions centered on a cry to understand how our loving God could allow such a lingering, miserable disease to continue among such caring, humble people.

Because of that trip, our nonprofit, *Love for Myanmar*, has expanded its ministry to include the Leprosy Hospital. Aside from an estimated 100 patients in the hospital, there is a nearby village of several hundred, mostly of their family members and a school of about sixty students. Because of the stigma of leprosy, there was no other place for these people to live. These ostracized Buddhists are in various degrees of spiritual decline and long for answers.

These people are facing a time of great discouragement and need the courage only available through our Lord, Jesus Christ. *Love for Myanmar* intends to share with these people how our Savior promises to love, protect, and guide us throughout our lives. None of us is immune to disappointment, struggles, and suffering. However, none of us need to face these challenges without hope. There is an answer!

God created both lepers and non-lepers; however, it is up to us Christians to figure out how we can best fit together. My time among the lepers has inspired a confidence that, despite their dark and distorted paths, they are interested in our spiritual views. What does that mean? It means they have come to trust the unconditional love which they have personally experienced from the hospital staff. This trust is unlocking their thinking to other ways of considering their future on earth—and afterwards.

The challenge is that they trust the staff's thinking, the staff's beliefs, but not their own about what the staff is sharing about Christianity. They believe the staff believes what the staff says they believe. It is like a child trusting a parent—not because they fully understand whatever the parent is sharing—but because they have come to trust the parent loves them and only has their best interest in mind.

I hope, *Love for Myanmar* will be able to aid the hospital staff by periodically bringing in caring people who can reinforce the staff's teachings, and help the patients develop their own foundation of understanding about Christianity and apply its truths to their daily lives. Our goal is to have each patient come to appreciate their unique identity and purpose, through an intimate relationship with Jesus Christ. With our efforts grounded in God's will, it is impossible to doubt its eventual success.

CHAPTER 5

✻

HOSPITAL GROUNDS

A man begins to die when he ceases to expect anything from tomorrow. -- ABRAHAM MILLER

THE CHRISTIAN LEPROSY HOSPITAL in Mawlamyine has been at the center of treating leprosy in Myanmar for over 100 years, chiefly because of the efforts of Susan Haswell. The daughter of James Haswell, who was an American Baptist missionary in Myanmar for over 40 years, Ms. Haswell became involved in one of the very first leper colonies, ensuring these people, who were banished to live in cemeteries, had food, shelter, and medicine. Her persistence resulted in the British government allowing her to purchase land affordably on which the lepers themselves, with their deformed hands, built the original structures in 1898.

As was the case throughout most of the history of leprosy, cultures treated the diseased mainly with the cowardly acts of isolation and ostracism. The very acts undertaken to protect populations perpetuated its existence by disgracing those whom it afflicted to the point of hiding their condition, beyond the reach of meaningful and timely treatment.

Today, on the same ground from which it began as a leper colony, the Christian Leprosy Hospital in Mawlamyine continues as a leprosy hospital, while also providing reconstructive surgery services and rehabilitation for people affected by leprosy. As a 100-bed facility with a 60-member staff, the Mawlamyine Leprosy Hospital is one of only two leprosy hospitals in Myanmar faced with serving an estimated population of 55 million people over a land area roughly the size of Texas.

The hospital exerts enormous influence over the property while embracing several other features within its compound, including a church, school, staff housing, and soccer field. Each feature is tethered to the other and shaped by their shared history and geography.

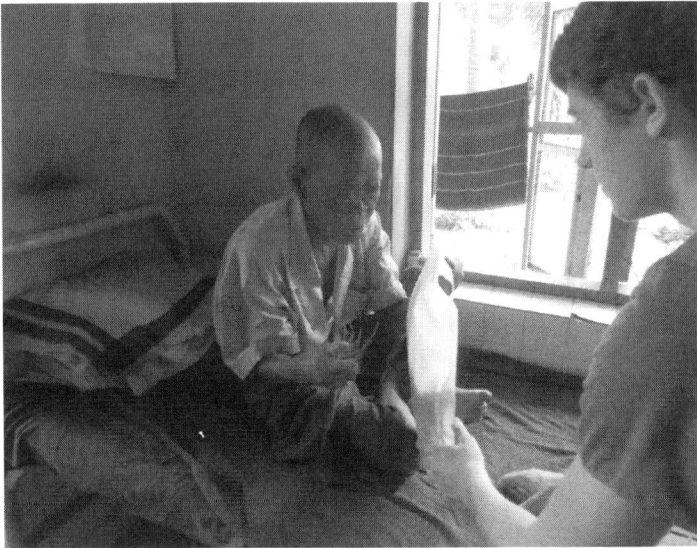

Collectively, there is an impersonal essence to the place, something that fails to account for the personalities within its boundaries, something that suppresses the human spirit. There is so much reality stuffed between the walls of these buildings the people dissolve into just identities.

That is, until you linger. After a while, you discover the tenderness, respect, patience, and thoughtfulness that is difficult to detect through a strange language, but recognizable through nonverbal ways—caring facial expressions, gentle laughter, and friendly embraces.

Nonetheless, all the compassion and love which the staff genuinely gives their patients cannot erase what it means to be called a leper. None of us has the slightest understanding of how that word permeates their hearts.

It was the condition of the buildings—inside and outside—that muzzled the truth about the goodness and harmony among the patients and staff. The drab, chipped ceilings and walls, dimly-lit and poorly-furnished rooms, narrow corridors and doorways, cramped offices and training spaces, together, suggested a cold, dark, inhumane place.

That partial truth cultivated an illusion that walled off, for a time, my ability to see the dichotomy of the hospital—its declining structures on the one hand and its impressive staff on the other.

Its run-down buildings continue to wither, creating a depressing environment for patients, staff, and visitors. The distressing surroundings compound the challenges for the staff, who remain unyielding in their collective pledge to serve the people under their care compassionately and professionally.

There is a church on the hospital grounds. It is a tired structure, resting just past a group of trees, toward the back of the property. It seems satisfied with allowing its age to run amuck with nature's elements, creating an unkept environment more suited to a rural setting. The congregation is mostly from the nearby Leprosy Village. As is the case in many churches in Myanmar, music is a key element in the Sunday worship service. Walls can be damaged, window glass broken, wooden pews splintered, cement floors cracked, but there will be an up-to-date sound system and musical instruments abounding. No matter the condition of the church building, its location, or the composition of the congregation, all the frustrations and sorrows of the week are overpowered by the passion which is expressed through the singing of its congregation.

Not too many steps from the church is a school. It is a pre-K school where little ones seem to be thinking, questioning, and imagining. Such open-mindedness and objectivity are uncommon in Myanmar where education is primarily based on recitation, and questions are viewed as disrespecting authority.

I suspect at such an early age your questions outnumber your knowledge, so you are less likely to be afraid of admitting not knowing something and more comfortable gathering answers. You could plop this group of about thirty young children from the Leprosy Village anywhere in an American pre-K school and they would do fine.

Three days a week some special education kids join the group. Although there is an occasional disruption, there are more instances where the special needs kids are helped voluntarily by the other children—sharing supplies, sharing floor space, sharing teachers. There is usually a territorial aspect that develops between students and teachers. Call it jealousy. I do not think even at this early age a child would allow another child to get closer to their teacher than he or she already is. When it happens, it is a testament to the loving environment created by the teachers.

Limited observation suggests the young village children are aware the other children are different but have decided the differences are negligible and simply relate from an instinct which recognizes another kind heart.

CHAPTER 6

LEPROSY DISEASE

I will never leave you nor forsake you. Hebrews 13:5 (NIV)

ALL AROUND THE WORLD, people go to their jobs, attend schools, and visit neighbors without the slightest thought of leprosy. Leprosy is a disease that, for most of us, is only found in medical journals as a reference to a once-feared infectious skin disease causing severe deformities and permanent disabilities. It has destroyed countless lives, not by killing the infected person, but through the resulting discrimination practiced by their home villages. Leprosy is curable and treatment in the early stages, through multi-drug therapy, can prevent disability.

However, Myanmar remains one of a handful of countries to be detecting thousands of new leprosy cases a year. Most of these cases involve patients from rural areas who simply are unfamiliar with the symptoms and have minimal access to a local health facility, causing unfortunate delays in treatment. Leprosy has been a public health problem in Myanmar for a very long time. The service area of the Leprosy Hospital in

Mawlamyine is mainly the Mon state, which has about three million people and is in southeastern Myanmar. The outpatient department treats thousands of patients each year, with most of these patients coming for the treatment of skin diseases.

It was the work of Dr. Armauer Hansen of Norway, in 1873, that provided unmistakable evidence that leprosy is caused by a germ, and not hereditary, a curse, or the result of sin.

The bacteria attacks nerve endings and destroys the body's ability to feel pain. As a result, people repeatedly injure themselves and the injuries become infected, which causes tissue loss. If left untreated, fingers can curl as small muscles are paralyzed, feet are damaged by unintended wounds and infection, and blindness can occur when facial nerves affect the blinking reflex of the eyes.

Generally, people suspected to have leprosy show symptoms such as pale or reddish patches on their skin, numbness or tingling of hands or feet, painful or tender nerves, and painless wounds or burns on hands or feet.

Although it is not fully understood how leprosy is spread, the consensus is the germ is transferred mainly by coughing and sneezing, through long-term contact with a person who has the disease but has not been treated. Most people will never develop the disease, as an estimated 95% of the world population has a natural immunity to leprosy.

Nonetheless, every two minutes someone around the world is diagnosed with leprosy, including about 150 people each year in the United States.

CHAPTER 7

HOSPITAL STAFF

Be steadfast, immovable, always abounding in the work of the Lord, knowing that in the Lord your labor is not in vain.
1Corinthians 15:58 (NIV)

CHRISTIANITY IS THE FOUNDATION ON which this hospital rests its identity, and the staff is its pillars, stabilizing the institution when doubts and fears mount from within its gates. All supervisory employees are Christian, while the non-supervisory positions are filled with former leprosy patients or family members who are mostly Buddhists.

The love and care of the staff for the patients is tiring, cursed with a multitude of other needs which continually drags the staff into a daily pit of exhaustion. Their compassion for the patients shows itself in their common, everyday interaction, but that is difficult to sustain under the relentless pressure of handling too many responsibilities for too little pay.

As a hospital staff person, the tension between the joy of believing you are doing something special as one of God's own and neglecting the basic needs of your own family is an ever-increasing difficulty. Understandably, passion has its price as younger staff leave for better wages.

It is challenging to have desperate people hold on to your words about hope when they have not experienced it, when they cannot see who you say can provide it, and when their view of your beliefs is limited to the uncertainty of their disease. Doctors and nurses can only stretch their patient's trust in them so far, as well as their trust in God to provide them with the spiritual confidence and composure to persevere with their efforts to share God's promises with the patients.

It takes extraordinary faith by the doctors and nurses, despite the patients' circumstances and despite minimal discernible results to intercede continually in the patients' lives, to refuse to allow their dark times to separate them from the promise of God's blessings.

Daily doctors, nurses, and other staff show evidence of God's grace to the patients and their families through their acts of genuine humility. They refuse to be indifferent about their patients' spirituality or judgmental about the drawbacks of their patients' religion.

They recognize the importance of hope to the state of the patient's mind and especially how its loss can penetrate the soul and distract the heart from caring about life—this one or the next. So, gently but persistently and each in their own way, not only carefully listens to understand the patients' lives, but tries to achieve an even greater understanding of what is specifically missing from those lives.

They see faces heavy with sorrow, they see souls filled with insecurity, and yet they continue to place themselves below their patients as humble servants confidently dependent on God. It is clear they have each given God the freedom to work within their respective hearts, which is why there remains the good possibility of making a difference in the lives of the patients around them.

Whatever progress the Mawlamyine Christian Leprosy Hospital has contributed toward sharing God's vision of the truth among the lepers and their families, rests with the hospital staff. I am not inclined to believe they just drifted together and landed at the hospital. As each took that step toward faithfully understanding where God was leading, their obedience placed them at this hospital.

The staff, both past and present, have their failings; however, their personal sacrifices, to be someone upon whom the patients can always count, are inspiring. However, it is an undermanned staff with an inadequate budget, working within an international health community preoccupied with more pressing priorities.

Most of the doctors' and nurses' work is hidden in every day conversations, normal routines, and common moments. It is as if they are always there, but invisible, except to that one patient they are beside.

To understand the Mawlamyine Christian Leprosy Hospital, you should understand its key staff. Here are their condensed stories, bound together by their commitment to the eternal well-being of their fellowman:

The Medical Superintendent

His parents are Christian and retired professionals—his father an economist at Yangon University, and his mother a civil engineer. Because of his high marks on the countrywide matriculation exam, he was placed in the medical profession track. Years later, on schedule, he graduated with his medical degree from Yangon University. In exchange for his free tuition from the government, he followed his graduation with three years of compulsory service in northern Myanmar. Ironically, years later, because of another doctor honoring his service commitment to the government, an opening occurred at the Leprosy Hospital in Mawlamyine, which he has filled since 2009. Now married, with a son and a daughter, he is the medical superintendent for the Mawlamyine Christian Leprosy Hospital.

He speaks softly and usually briefly. He has a gift for being insightful without elaboration. However, there are times when you sense he is scanning your brain, eavesdropping on your thoughts, to be sure you are not disappointed with him. His calm manner belies the intensity of his caring concern for his patients and their family members, as well as his staff and their family members. He has an unassuming presence, engaging smile, and sincerity in his tone that reflects his affection, devotion, and reverence for the hospital.

To most bystanders, I am sure this hospital is just a building, but I am convinced that for him, it is where his heart calls home.

The Ex-Hospital Board Member

Unique background; unique experiences; unique person— these words highlight this doctor-turned-freelance consultant and ex-hospital board member. Born in the Mon state, she was raised in a Christian home by a father who was a small businessman and a mother who was a nurse. Despite being Baptists, her parents sent her to a Catholic convent in Mawlamyine because of its recognition as a high quality educational institution. As a result, she saw her parents and six other siblings infrequently.

With a medical degree from the Institute of Medicine I, Yangon, she was with the Department of Health of the Government of Myanmar for almost twenty years. She left the country to work in Ethiopia for thirteen years, which included a stint as an UN volunteer, then with UNICEF, and finally with the African Medical and Research Foundation. She returned home to Myanmar in 2003, doing freelance work, especially in the field of HIV/AIDS. She served the Mawlamyine Christian Leprosy Hospital as a board member from 2006 to 2014. Currently, she is working with the hospital to develop a fifteen-year business plan that, by the grace of God, shall not only "bring greater glory to His name" but also, as a Myanmar praise and worship song goes, "let everyone in Myanmar know about Christ."

Conversations with her are like fireside chats. Her casual style of communicating, coupled with her charming disposition, creates transparency—a refreshing openness in a culture where pleasing the other party is often placed above the truth. She thinks, feels, and acts, focused only on the best interests of the hospital, and as a result, leaves you with an lasting awareness of what bringing glory to God truly means.

The Matron

Her father, who was a Baptist pastor, regularly visited the leprosy patients and encouraged her to help at the hospital. He was straightforward with her about the risks involved, but also about being fulfilled when serving "the least of these." She embraced her father's advice and has grown an admirable legacy.

Her heart must be ninety percent of her body. She pumps out love at an astonishing rate, indiscriminately, throughout the day. Although a small woman, her presence, which is a blend of compassion, practicality, and wisdom, towers over the day's challenges. For over thirty years at this hospital, she has listened and counseled thousands about their hopes and fears, their struggles with relationships, and their anguished searches for answers to this unfortunate twist in their lives.

No small part of her job is comforting the emotionally wounded and trying to answer the questions that inevitably rise from becoming a leper.

She values people and, most of all, Jesus Christ. As she walks along the hospital's corridors and the pathways on the property, I think this place fills her soul beyond her father's expectations.

CHAPTER 8

LEPROSY VILLAGE

Hope does not disappoint. Romans 5:5 (NIV)

THE NEARBY VILLAGE isn't a village...it's a warehouse. It is where, despite signed agreements between the hospital and their families to take them back, cured patients continue to try to make it. It is where ordinary living is uncommon. It's where the past is overvalued, and futures are underestimated. It is where even cured patients cannot find jobs locally. Being cured is only the beginning of this disease.

It's where the dimensions of relationships are measured only by the depth of shared despair. No jobs, no money, no future... it is that simple. Their frustration justified. Their escape unlikely. Each wait for the other's tears to dry, wondering what is to become of them.

It's where an eerie calm covers the days, hiding the worst of diseases—loneliness.

The fact that this village exists is an unfortunate contradiction. From this geographic box, which traces its origin to the worst of mankind's ways—prejudice, hostility, injustice, in-dignity—arises a host of humble, forgiving, peaceful, upright people. Cruelly forced from their home villages, disowned by their families, shamed by their religion, these people gradu-ally came together forging their own community. Unlike other places, everyone knows why everyone else is here. They share the same core story. There are no hidden motives, power struggles, or disguised self-interests. It may be the most transparent place on earth. These lepers, these outcasts, these "low lives" have risen above the forces of deceit, revenge, and pity that ensnare the rest of us.

CHAPTER 9

※

FIRST IMPRESSIONS

As he thinks in his heart, so is he. Proverbs 23:7 (NIV)

ON MY WAY TO THE CITY of Mawlamyine, the capitol of the Mon state and the location of the Leprosy Hospital, every mile became its own unique frame. Every frame presenting a different shade of green. The unceasing rain never seems to tire of playing with the green. After all, it is the monsoon season.

During the monsoon season (typically May through October), everything in Myanmar moves. There is a vitality among nature brought on by the kind of rain that occurs in few places on this earth. You are encouraged to dismiss most of this movement as your curiosity will usually lead to alarm over the never-ending small creatures (ants, bugs, lizards) continually trying to reclaim their territory from the season. Myanmar is dripping with life.

In a string of 30 to 45-second bursts, the intensity of the rain is as if God is playing with a switch in the heavens causing the rain from above to reach out to the rain already fallen, lifting the ground's horizon beyond my experiences. There is no place the rain cannot reach as vegetation even grows, at all angles, out of the mixture of plastic sheeting, brick, tin, bamboo, whatever was available at the time of a building's construction. Tree branches jut peculiarly from the side of businesses, as if lost, looking for soil they won't find at two or three stories high. You can hear the branches' panicked conversations, wondering how they got to where they are, and where they go from here. "Damn rain. I should have never allowed my thirst such freedom."

The landscape is a mixture of sporadic progress whispering in the ear of centuries-old traditions to "move aside"—cell towers emerging from paddy fields, neon signs blinking colorful advertisements over dull brown bamboo huts, and modern air-conditioned buses like mine wrestling for space with aged motorbikes carrying entire families over narrow, unstriped roadways.

As I made my way beyond the hospital's weathered sign and then through its molded arch, my eyes were presented with a building that had been treated unkindly by the climate and, even worse, by time. You could see all its one hundred plus years of life staring back at you through its discolored, blotched, and wrinkled face of painted walls. Before you stepped onto its ground, you knew there was something different about this place; something its history wanted to say.

I was surprised by the hospital's location. I was thinking it would be a healthy distance from the city...isolated, remote. However, there it was, nestled inside the city's boundaries, resting wearingly among neighborhoods, trying to gain a new respect for its work while protecting itself from the misguided perspectives of its past. I discovered the hospital was originally outside the city; however, the tentacles of the city have gradually encircled the compound, preying on its future by squeezing the soul from its past.

This hospital building's aged walls are like the pages of a special, worn book—the edges are soft, the binding struggles to hold, but the story remains intact when we are willing to turn the pages with care.

Walking around inside, there was an uncommon quietness where somberness rested on the air, weighing down any optimism. There was staff passing from one area to another and an occasional family member finding their way to their loved one's bedside. However, there was something missing amid this activity. There was no joy in anyone's greeting. There was no passion in anyone's conversation. There was no purpose in anyone's walk. There was no promise on anyone's face.

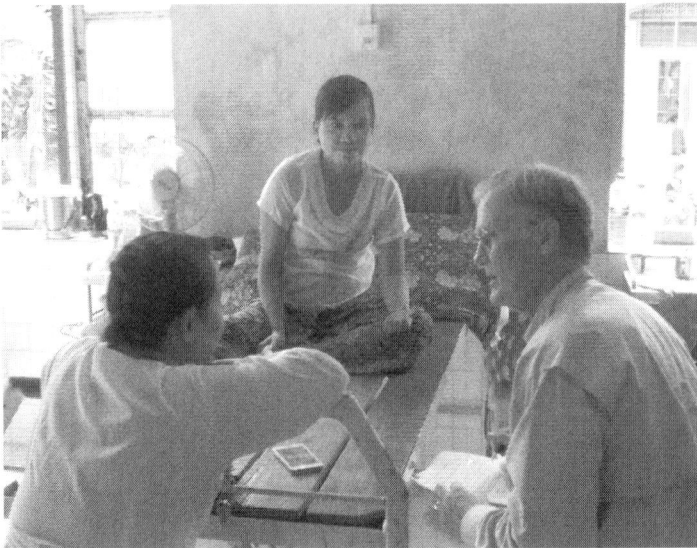

Although there are seven wards, including separate female and male medical and surgical wards, there are no private patient rooms. There are just common areas where patients are grouped by the dozen and their privacy defined by their wooden-slatted bed, small table stand, and plastic stool.

However, most of their time is lived in the room within the room-the room of "religious deception" where your disease is considered punishment, your treatment is considered a waste of resources, and your recovery is considered solely your responsibility. Each day, from this room, they surrender their hope believing whatever bad decisions they have made in their lives have conspired against them and led to their present unsurmountable unhappiness.

It was from within this inner room that I found myself visiting with them—lepers who felt unworthy of my time and who believed themselves to be beyond any god's compassion.

CHAPTER 10

LEPROSY PATIENTS

Comfort and prosperity have never enriched the world as much as adversity has. -- *BILLY GRAHAM*

I BEGAN STARING at the hospital walls, and that is when the building's history broke its silence. It hadn't deteriorated because of the weather battering its outside walls. It was gradually being overcome by the sadness within its walls. Year after year, it has watched patients lying in their beds, hour upon hour, with no sense of direction about their future.

Many a patient's tear laced face has turned to its walls searching for answers about why their lives had placed them here. Patients' deformed hands have reached out in the night and touched its walls in desperation to feel something in return. Patients would often stare at the ceiling from their beds, whispering question after question about their suffering to someone—someone they have never met, someone whose name they do not know, but someone they hoped was there.

They seem as if they have allowed their circumstances to convince them they are "nobodies." Most of us need to learn from someone, other than a family member, that we are known, we are loved, and we are not alone. To whom can they turn for encouragement, truth, or courage? In whom can they confide when they wonder what others think when looking at their deformities?

This isn't the life they had imagined or wanted. Oh, how they wish they could go back to a simpler time, a time when their future hadn't so much mystery. Maybe they were never meant to be complete, maybe they were never meant to chase dreams. This earth is seldom a kind place for lepers.

Their disease caused them to lose their way while joy has passed them by. One day's pain spills over into the next. There's no place it cannot reach. It's always by their side, holding on to the shattered pieces of the life they once knew. There are no words to explain why they don't live that life any more. Who can possibly pull them through the shadows of their despair, get them to believe their story is not finished, and walk them beyond the hospital's door? There is more beyond their heartache, beyond their scars, beyond their tears.

They live in the past, in a time before their disease. Their idea of the future is unformed and much shorter than the past to which they desperately cling. They are giving up any joy in this life by allowing their despair to harden their hearts. It is like watching death come alive! Listless and exhausted from a condition of hopelessness that penetrates their spirit for life and weakens their will, they gradually let go of the smallest whispers of joy.

They are understandably ungrateful for this life and live among those who also keep the deep wounds of their hearts as promises to themselves never to forgive life for their difficulty. They cannot change on their own because they don't understand their scars!

It is unbelievable how a leper's life is less about their physical afflictions and more about their spiritual torment. Medications have been developed specifically to treat leprosy, and they are effective—leprosy is curable. Regrettably, it metastasizes itself, through the prejudiced actions of others, to the patient's soul. Hearts become jaundiced, attitudes become caustic, and wills become weak.

Their Bond

Greater love has no one than this, that someone lay down his life for his friends. John 15:13 (NIV)

There are times when the patients help one another resurrect childhood memories—memories which have a grip on their hearts to a happier time. These patches of beauty periodically decorate their minds but struggle for space to stretch beyond a few moments. Inevitably, they quickly descend back to the darkness of their day, unchanged, feeling like a leper again.

If change is ever to come, it will begin through their fellow patients, each of whom uniquely contributes to an environment where fears, doubts, and struggles can be safely expressed. It's where each helps the other to engineer their circumstances, risking it all for moments of genuine, wondrous understanding.

It is pleasing to be able to abandon yourself and be among those who feel no pity about your deficiencies and speak honestly from their hearts. It is this honesty which provides the light by which they help one another see the fullness of their uniqueness.

There seems to be a common language among the patients, a quiet attentiveness within a tangled network of relationships that threads itself honorably throughout each day. Crisscrossing the room, hundreds of times a day, are the tiniest of connections, the nearly invisible yet extraordinarily meaningful messages exchanged among patients—nods of understanding, gestures of encouragement, glimpses of empathy.

This isolation, their respective loneliness, reinforces their reliance on one another to construct another world, a reality that works for them. They share the heart-wrenching silence of waiting together to see no visitors—again. Then, when the rest of the world is sleeping, they are alert and attentive to one another's cries. When the few relatives leave their side, they protect one another from the harmful loneliness which enters its own way.

Somehow, in an atmosphere of loneliness, a sense of community emerges; a camaraderie brought on by their shared disease but nurtured by their need for human understanding; a camaraderie that allows the truth about themselves to be shown among themselves; a camaraderie that keeps them from being pulled into the depths of despair by the weight of their own experiences.

They want their truth to escape, their feelings to be known, their perspective on their world to be shared, to go anywhere but where it is now. Now, it just gets routinely passed among themselves, eventually resting on their instincts to accept their circumstances calmly and trust few beyond the borders of their disease.

This protective coating of understanding that has formed over the patients has made the decision to return home to the unknown less desirable. Why subject yourself to more pain?

What is a friend? A single soul dwelling in two bodies. --
ARISTOTLE

Individual Stories

Do not pray for easy lives. Pray to be stronger men. Do not pray for tasks equal to your powers. Pray for powers equal to your tasks. Then the doing of your work shall be no miracle, but you shall be the miracle. -- PHILLIPS BROOKS

On entering the ward, each patient watches you impassively; lost beyond the need of the moment. Nothing on the other side of their room's walls seems of the slightest interest. They prefer to loiter in their minds, allowing their suffering to speak for them, while they blend into the hospital's landscape.

For sure, their scars are deep and push tomorrows far away. Although the clouds of their sorrow gathered during our time together, they still tried to reach across the years to share their hurts with me.

They admitted to toying with reintroducing themselves to their villages, only to discover an ignorance about their disease that had grown oblivious to the psychological torture it inflicted. Where does the blame for this stagnated view of a curable disease rest? In part, it can be credited to the tragic irony there are hundreds of villages found beyond the reach of any hospital or medical clinic, and it is these places from which the new cases of leprosy arise. With few exceptions, villagers make their way to legitimate caregivers only after enduring intensive periods of puzzling changes to their bodies or being forcibly isolated from their communities because of diagnoses grounded in uninformed fear and arbitrary tradition.

Another unfortunate contributing cause is their fellow Buddhists, who continually intimidated these sufferers into accepting responsibility for their disease. In the name of protecting their religion, families, friends, and others are demonstrating a decreasing toleration for lepers trying to reinsert themselves into their respective villages. With their basic support network decimated, lepers have been shamed into subjugating their own best health interests, and thereby have defaulted to the position that they deserve to be disfigured or crippled.

When I look into their faces and learn their stories, I cannot imagine being able to help them find joy in their condition, purpose in their deformity, and hope in the direction their suffering can take them. It feels cruel to continue.

Nonetheless, somehow these people have found their way into my heart, and while I grip the railing of my grief for them, I will share some of the fragments of their stories.

It was challenging to assemble the pieces of their stories before my own emotion produced its own pain. Occasionally, I was helpless to take notes while drifting in and out of conversations, untethered with any purpose other than just listening. Their words poured right through me—simple to my mind and sweet to my heart—as I surrendered my hands to my side and took notes on my opened heart.

What began as a well-intended attempt to capture the stories of lepers and, hopefully, bring awareness of their struggles to others, seemed more like intrusions into the tender spots of their pain. I am under no illusion that they have mastered sharing with outsiders only what allows them to move their focus away from their circumstance temporarily. Nonetheless, I tried to disarm their anxiety, but no amount of planning can fully bring teetering apprehension back from the edge of privacy.

Their courage of mind to share blended with my charity of soul to serve and overcame their wish to be left alone and my guilt for intruding on their privacy.

Together we sought the boundary of sharing, marshaled our mutual respects, and proceeded with the delicate exploration of a leper's life. I hope, God will use their sharing to awaken a desire in you to be a genuine extension of God's love to them. Leprosy is an overreaching disease that repeatedly

claims parts of people's lives who are not directly infected. Loneliness and hopelessness are unfortunate obstacles to recovery, and the truth about a cure is a frequent casualty to cultural and religious preferences.

Living in dignity, free from the abuse and neglect which threatens every leper, is a prized goal and one the hospital tries to achieve, despite its limitations.

Consider this fifty-something couple. At age 12, her pastor brought her to the Leprosy Hospital. She had been forced from her village and was living with her grandmother; a two-hour walk through the jungle. At the hospital, she met another young patient and over the following six years, their relationship culminated into marriage—he was 20, she 18.

As patients, the hospital hired them to work in the kitchen while living in the nearby village. They were hospital employees for 15 years, converted from Buddhism to Christianity, and have raised six children. They attend the church on the leprosy grounds where he serves as a deacon.

The perceived threats of leprosy did not crush these two people. The hospital staff knew well the risks confronting this couple and dared to defend their cure against the usual abandonment of society. Their success is a vivid example of the emptiness of thoughts built around the premise that lepers are unequal citizens who are incapable of contributing productively to our world.

There is nothing about her life she owns. She has given up everything to this disease. It explains to her what each day will bring. She doesn't have any relationships that can compete with it—except her 12-year-old daughter who is sitting by her side on the bed.

She is a beautiful young girl, no longer in school, who in many respects has become responsible for her mother. There is something purposeful behind that gaze toward me, something that reassured me her mom was in good hands. There is no doubt that each belongs completely to the other, each delight in being with the other.

Suffering from a reaction to the treatments, this mid-thirty-aged woman is severely jaundiced, and is now trying to recuperate from a different set of medicines. Her body appears tired, and her soul seems exhausted.

She doesn't want to return to her village. By manipulating the fear of leprosy, her mother-in-law has turned everyone against her, taken over the household, and relegated her to servant status in her own home. The bitterness, hostility, and isolation within her own home and village have become intolerable.

Yet, she considers her current situation an opportunity, a chance to consider other options, without having to deal with the constant jabs to her self-worth. So, here she is—a recovering leper whose husband is unemployed, whose oldest daughter is not in school, whose 3 1/2-year-old daughter is under the care of a misguided mother-in-law, and whose future rests on a fragile spirit clearly at a turning point.

Since the age of 14, he has either lived in the hospital as a patient or in the nearby Leprosy Village as an outcast from his home village. As he learned some years later, the doctor advised him that in the beginning, he had a skin condition and not leprosy. The thinking at the time was to try to stretch this teenager's stay at his home village, to experience a normal life among family and friends, for as long as possible. While under treatment and not contagious, he wore long-sleeve shirts and eventually masks cut from towels for his face to hide the sores which covered his body.

Realizing the Leprosy Hospital was noted for its expertise in treating various skin ailments, villagers did not consider his trips to their facility alarming.

Nonetheless, as his periodic visits to the Leprosy Hospital mounted, so did the concern among the villagers that he was being regularly exposed to leprosy, could become infected, and risk the health of the village.

Their concern eventually culminated into a demand that until his condition was cured, he could not return to the village. He has not returned in over 50 years!

Long ago cured of leprosy, he is married with grandchildren and retired as a longtime hospital employee. Along the way, after about seven years with the hospital, he converted to Christianity and has since led each of his family members to Jesus Christ as well.

His story should cause us to wonder how we would respond to such a situation. When circumstances are engineered in such a challenging way, what will it reveal about our character?

Imagine having your life so drastically changed at the age of fourteen and to think you are of no value to anyone, to forget whatever dreams you had, to realize that those closest to you can no longer be relied on for support. The battle is on you. There is no time to prepare. In order not to jeopardize your loved ones, you hide your feelings, take a glance at the life which will no longer be possible, and leave for a future with an unseen course.

Each of us must ask ourselves, how did we get to where we are and what do we want to leave behind? Some of us will collapse under the weight of the questions, while others will conquer their fear and be open to all God can be in our next moments.

Each of us wants to be the best we can be, to be transformed into that person we are designed to be. However, few of us willingly place ourselves in circumstances that will demand from us the exercising of our responsibility for our own spiritual renewal. We are accountable for placing our faith in action, for recognizing that each day is just one piece of God's plan for us to be honored with our best effort.

✺

Life was a struggle but manageable. Her husband could usually find work in the patty fields or as a gardener. Earnings were not much but enough to ensure their daughters were healthy. At age 40, she had not expected more and had settled into the present where she devoted her time, energy, and interest to caring for her family.

Most days ended in contented exhaustion, and then there was that night. The night her body was telling her something she simply did not understand. Over the following weeks, the strange changes to her skin caused her thinking to go from being puzzled to being alarmed.

However, there was no medical clinic anywhere close to their village. Months passed and being able to shroud her condition became increasingly difficult.

Under the guise of visiting her sister, she made her way to Yangon. Exhausted from the secrecy, she cautiously shared her situation with her sister. Her desperation was rewarded as the friendship of their hearts brought tears of oneness to their faces. Later that week, because of a doctor's examination, her suspicions were confirmed. She had leprosy.

Since that time nearly two years ago, she has received the correct treatments, however, her body has been reacting negatively to the drug therapy. She is undergoing different treatments with no idea about her future.

***

Time and again, patients throw themselves on the mercy of their home villages, only to learn that walls have been built up through ignorance about their disease—an ignorance that denies the healing and freedom years of treatment offer. This is a unique social ill whose root of ignorance runs deep through the generations and traps villagers in a web of insecurity from which they seldom escape.

Gradually, out of a sense of frustration, patients lay aside their dreams of going back to their villages and reuniting with their families and surrender to the bondage of hopelessness.

Most of their relationships have been disconnected at the other end—where families and friends once were. Every patient has their own story about how communications were cut off, visits disappeared, and phone calls unanswered. The paradox is how absence becomes a presence, silence becomes a sound, and loneliness becomes a friend.

As I approached the doorway to leave the hospital and looked back, this place made one last powerful statement: The Lord has not forgotten these people; He is here among them. It is us, who profess to be Christians, who are the true unfortunates to be forgotten by the Lord as He watches us pass by those in need.

Unfortunately, we proudly make more of our presence in such a place as this hospital than we make of His presence in us. It is His presence in us that will change their hearts, change their eternity.

Lepers are a visible reminder of the presence of God in our midst, not His absence. They should remind us of our blessings and our commitments to love others without fear. When we leave them behind, we are abandoning the Christian principles we claim to believe...we are leaving behind, God. And, with every step taken away, we draw nearer to an empty future filled with the mystery of not knowing what God could have done through us and the unfortunate realization that we are seldom as good as we think.

CHAPTER 11

RELIGIOUS PERSPECTIVES

Whoever knows the right thing to do and fails to do it, for him it is sin. James 4:17 (NIV)

OVER THE YEARS, it has been shared with me that "to be Burmese is to be Buddhist." There is an unquestioned bond throughout the country between the religion and the people of Myanmar. Buddhism is ingrained in the national identity.

While an estimated 90% of the people in Myanmar are Buddhists, 100% of the patients in the Leprosy Hospital are Buddhists. There is no way to gauge their devoutness, so we are proceeding with the understanding that they embrace the core teachings of Buddhism, that life is full of suffering, which is a result of unfilled desires—owning things, enjoying things. The goal of a devout Buddhist is to free yourself from your desires because they cause your suffering. The quantity and quality of your "good deeds" (what you think, say, and do) impacts your level of suffering, which influences your status in your next life. Each person is on their own to find their way from one life to the next. There are no gods nor saviors on whom to rely for guidance. Indeed, devotion to any god can only lead to disappointment, confusion, and sorrow.

Being Buddhist, there is a distance between themselves and God. They are living scared in the shadows, with no sense of God's presence, where trusting that their suffering will end is increasingly difficult.

I sense there is a deepening understanding among the patients that there is more to this life and beyond than their current religion can handle. They are more aware that their spiritual lives are stagnant, that the quality of their inner journey is no longer acceptable. There is an increasing awareness that the truth, not about their disease but about life itself, has been kept from them, that their religion has abandoned them to the consequences of their circumstances. They and their religion have grown sad together.

In my judgment, their minds are on auto pilot using the language of "cultural tradition" because that's the most comfortable approach to take if you value your social freedom. They have allowed themselves to become dominated by philosophical beliefs and practices passed between generations, which silence questions about Christianity while leading to the atrophy of critical thinking about Buddhism.

The patient's physical condition is intimately connected to their spiritual mind-set, which has led them to assume they are unworthy of anyone's touch. They are "paying twice" by allowing their affliction to distort their perception of other people—thinking everyone else is perfect, while they are imperfect; thinking everyone else lives a normal life, while they are not part of this world; thinking everyone else has relationships, while they are separated from them. The inescapable absence of normalcy, unfortunately, keeps their longings for genuine intimacy hidden.

The patients' hearts are not hardened toward God. There is no shell that's formed around their understanding of Jesus Christ. They are sadly drifting from one false promise to another within the only spiritual environment they have ever known. They are preoccupied with things that have little or no eternal value. They are enmeshed in a spiritual life that is deceiving them and causing them to trust innocently in matters which distance them from the one true God.

Most of their lives have been defined with no knowledge of God, no awareness of the Bible, no understanding of Christian community in Myanmar.

I think some of them would be willing learners, open to being taught by God through their suffering. However, no one is taking the time to help them place their struggles in a Godly context. To consider that their situation has a purpose, their suffering has meaning, their brokenness can be a blessing is unimaginable. Who among us will humble themselves to open the gates to the presence of God for these lepers?

Perhaps your experiences can be the beginning of the change in them. Perhaps your time there can be the beginning of the discovery you are seeking in yourself.

It is difficult to imagine a more chilling scene than people standing at grace's archway, would-be believers, so close to hope and glory, being swept into hell—their journey stopped at heaven's gates by our unwillingness to let God be all He can be in us.

They are holding on to where they think they belong. Their heart-wrenching experiences have not made God real, only that they deserve the disease they have. You are not being asked to help erase the memories of their ordeals. You are being asked to have them consider there is a purpose for their suffering and hope beyond their pain.

It feels to me like Myanmar's lepers are in a strange place. Their unhappiness is toxic to their well-being, and yet, their unhappiness is tied to their religion, which has bent their will inward toward guilt rather than outward to embrace understanding. Rather than draw purpose from their unsettling condition through their religion, they are left to handle the gravity of their circumstance alone. Not to be threatening but realistic, be mindful that, although their religion is formidable, it is not invincible. We must balance two competing realities—Buddhism, which rejects the existence of a Creator God and the soul, and Christianity, which teaches there is one God who we are to love wholeheartedly.

For me, these competing realities can best be illustrated as differing lights. Buddhism is a blinding light shining in your face, brightening only itself. Christianity is a guiding light shining from beside you, revealing the path ahead of you and escorting you to your destination.

I sense a thirst among the lepers for a purpose behind their suffering, for people (of courage) to help them heal their spiritual wounds. We need to turn our minds back to those times when the currents of powerlessness swept through our own lives and challenged those beliefs we held dear.

In Myanmar, we may find ourselves on a spiritual island, unconnected to anyone, isolated with these lepers, drifting together, thankfully, farther from the shores of bias, criticism, and fear. This generation of lepers can enrich the lives of those following, as well as their families, if we can even lightly imprint on their hearts and souls the beautiful truth of our God's care, kindness, and love for them.

For sure, there will be a cost to sharing alternative religious viewpoints, offering different moral choices, and providing a more truthful approach to eternity. However, as Christians, we cannot allow this situation to be defined by our silence.

CHAPTER 12

PERSONAL
REFLECTIONS

Christian communities across Burma (Myanmar) continue to experience deep pain and suffering, due to egregious violations of religious freedom. RACHEL FLEMING, HIDDEN PLIGHT: CHRISTIAN MINORITIES IN BURMA

WHAT FOLLOWS IS A COLLECTION of my thoughts as jotted down at various times throughout my journey. I am unsure they will have any meaning beyond their lettering. Nonetheless, they represent my thinking at that time.

I was standing at my hotel room window gazing out to a world that both mystified and saddened me when I began to wonder:

The hospital has an address, but its patients do not—no cards, no letters, no packages, no visits. Is it because their families and friends do not know where they are? Or, is it because they know exactly where they are? They forced them to the hospital; away from the one address they did not want them to have—their own.

Always hidden in the shadows of other's ignorance, neglected from hour to hour, the lepers' only satisfaction come

50

when the night nudges the day aside. I think they delight in the darkness because it shields them from their misery; a unique disease that you can see march on your body, while knowing it cares nothing about the life it disfigures.

It seems loneliness has a way of whispering to these isolated souls only about their disabilities, to blind them from even imagining themselves living productively in our world. Such conversations have built a relationship with loneliness that has guided their will to dwell only on their inadequacies. On another occasion, I was lying in the hotel bed shifting toward the light from the lamp on the nightstand, which my tiredness had neglected to turn off, when I began to wonder:

What will become of these men and women with leprosy? How many of them simply want to be swallowed up by this earthly life, never again to feel abandoned, hopeless, and worthless?

For just a moment, imagine yourself in their bodies. Would such a daily condition wear you down and rob you of all hope? Would you share your sorrow? Would you call your circumstance a life? For how long could you endure the desertion of family and friends?

Indifference to leprosy is a disease within a disease. Leprosy affects every ethnicity and culture and impacts developing countries like Myanmar more harshly. Where is the hope? In whom can they trust their sorrow? To whom can they turn to protect their soul against the assaults of ostracism and

misunderstanding, which regularly robs them of companion-
ship and compassion?

※

Whether sitting in the dark, at a table in the early morning, waiting for the restaurant staff to set out breakfast or from a cracked
plastic chair placed in the corner of a sidewalk café, with the
blurred image of a monk chanting from an aged television, my
mind would drift between bites and sips into wondering:

Is our concern for these lepers counterfeit? Are we just
creating comfortable opportunities of service, which require
minimal sacrifice, while claiming to be someone we have
never been?

It seems we spend much of our lives protecting ourselves from
challenges which could position us to experience God's blessings.

It is occurring to me that it is not the disease which prevents
us from helping these lepers, it is our failure to try to understand
genuinely the purpose their hardship has in God's plan for us.

Surely, these people were never meant to carry such a load
by themselves, and yet, there is no one beside them, resulting
in no one inside them. Their emptiness is indulging in our absence. Their suffering is an opportunity to serve those pre-
cious in His sight and a privilege to add dignity to our own
lives. I believe God has written something on each of our
hearts, the pursuit of which will lead to mutual enrichment
for us and especially those we serve.

But, for reasons which never seek God's insights, we ig-
nore the tug of God's promises and embrace instead the comfort of lives of our own making.

I pray each of us will take the initiative to run our thoughts along the words of fulfillment God has engraved on our hearts and pour out His life-changing love to the patients, families, and staff of the leprosy community in Mawlamyine.

Christians are not immune from feelings of pride, from flattering ourselves when we have suffered for our faith. We get too preoccupied with wanting the world to see the evidence of our impact, rather than being internally satisfied when our obedience has brought joy to our God's heart.

Where is the outward expression of our inward knowledge of God's love? Where are the Christians to help them not remove their sorrow, but understand it? Where are the Christians on whom these people can count for encouragement, to draw on for spiritual guidance, to provide an assurance they are loved?

Then, there were the hours spent traveling—by bus from Yangon to the Mon state, by truck from Mawlamyine to Hpa-an, by bus back to Yangon and, of course, the airplane rides from and to the United States through Tai Pei to Myanmar. Time which found me regularly arguing, questioning, defending myself as a leper to my Christian self. A typical session went something like this:

Leper: Why should I believe what you say? You will soon be getting on a plane. Why would I want to know about a loving God who has surrounded me with so much sorrow? What makes you think I would believe in the promises of your God, the God who allows such a disease to scar my life?

Me: Inside the hospital, I did not sense even the hum of another civilization. The thickness of the patients' mistrust of the outside world rivals the thickness of the walls in which you find yourselves, resulting in little curiosity beyond the view some of you have from your dusty windows. It is as if such glimpses are punishments, reminders of a life you now consider beyond your reach. You have crafted an approach to life that tries to minimize any distractions, messages, or memories from your previous life. You have adeptly harnessed your suffering into an ever-increasing condition of self-imposed depression.

Leper: We have come to understand what you call depression as trying to draw hope from a never-ending well of doubt. What is the point to being declared "cured" if we cannot get jobs, if we cannot find housing, if we cannot develop relationships? The outside world is a battlefield strewn with land mines that eventually are too exhausting for us to navigate.

Me: You just get caught in the relentless swirl of despair inside your heads and gradually seclude yourselves from others, inviting only "your kind" to share the intimacy of your hurts. You're entangled in fear, which has become an all-consuming condition of your lives. This fear has drawn an artificial boundary around each day, creating a snare in which hope disappears. We should force your fear to come face-to-face with our God's love.

Leper: While doctors can improve our health circumstances, they cannot heal the wounds of isolation. You have no idea what the "silence of hope" is like. We gain a fondness for being lonely. We flood ourselves with hurtful self-talk, to crowd out being hurt by others. There is an unrelenting curiosity of "why me." No matter where we are or what we are doing, there is no such thing as a cured leper.

How can we have faith in something, if we are unaware of its existence? How can we challenge our present beliefs, if there is nothing which shows itself more trustworthy? We know what we have. We know the treatment options. We know the probable outcomes. Few of us struggle with the medical realities. It is the exposure to the nonmedical realities which overpower us and hold us captive.

We have become prisoners clinging to our own chains of fear, sorrow, and worthlessness, pacing about a future in which we are missing.

Several times I felt my mind climb over itself to get a better view of all I had experienced. With a second wind, I appealed to my awkward, muffled sense of shame and fear about lepers, trying to get my brain to trust what my experiences indented on my heart. And, my wondering continued:

How can my God be who I believe Him to be while allowing such suffering? This hospital is a place where my God could do great works. Then, I realize that true to His word, God IS here. He is just alone.

What have I done to honor my debt to God? I know God is there, we are just not conversant because my unwillingness to accept my responsibility as a Christian, to give these lepers a chance at knowing my God, has placed my own spirituality in doubt.

As a result, I continue to deal with my own ostracism—where my best intentions to help, continue to be banished to a remote corner of my soul. What I am feeling is the frustration of being unable to connect the genuine loneliness of these lepers with the genuine love of my God. Isn't the evidence of our beliefs in the hope it provides?

These lepers have no idea the influence they are having on my spirituality. There is no conscious attempt on their behalf to move me to act. They are like stars silently positioned in the distant sky, in their place, mostly taken for granted, until the intensity of their sorrow pierces holes in my faith. Has my Christianity become defined by the distance from which they are from my world or my distance from God?

What is considered sacrifice? When God is unknown to you, is the fact that you have leprosy considered a sacrifice? Is a disease just a form of meaningless suffering, if you have no spiritual context in which to place it? Can these lepers be led to understand that their suffering is an expression of love, designed by their Creator to draw them closer to an everlasting relationship with Him?

How do you persuade someone, such as a leper, to believe in the healing properties of suffering? From where, from whom will such a breakthrough come?

How can we STAND BY and expect unbelievers to handle their situation without knowing Jesus Christ?

How can we PASS BY and expect unbelievers to understand their future without knowing God has a plan for it?

How can we say GOODBYE and expect unbelievers to know there is more than pain and suffering in this life without sharing the hope and love of Jesus Christ?

And then, there was the dream. The dream that snuck up on me, while napping, on my airplane ride home.

I have but one candle of life to burn, and I would rather burn it out in a land filled with darkness than a land flooded with light. -- JOHN KEITH FALCONER

It began with a picture of a candle burning in the darkness, followed by images showing a busy, active, happy man fully engaged in Myanmar's rural life. Images rolled by of various village scenes—young men playing soccer, villagers gathered for a meal, people visiting along the dirt paths.

Then, the man spoke: "I'm exhausted. I've got to pace myself. I'm involved in too many activities. I just don't have enough time for my family or myself. I enjoy these outings with my friends. I always look forward to the village gatherings and the storytelling after sharing a meal. The pick-up soccer games, the spur-of-the-moment ventures into the nearby big village, the drop-in visits to my friends' houses; they are all enjoyable, but I've got to manage my time better. I'm neglecting my guitar playing, and I haven't finished that landscape painting for my Mom."

Then he is awakened. "Mr. Htoo, Mr. Htoo. It's time for your session. Do you hear me? Are you awake?"

The man resumes talking: "I lean on the nurse's shoulder as she guides me toward the therapy room. The walk is slow and painful. We could certainly use more wheelchairs."

The session ends, and so ends the day. There's still plenty of daylight. There's still plenty of time remaining in the day. There's just nothing to fill the time.

There are no drop-in visits from family or friends. There are no pick-up games or spur-of-the-moment guitar jam sessions.

I'm exhausted, but not from being overwhelmed with activities. I'm exhausted from being overwhelmed by my feelings of hopelessness and loneliness which comes from being a leper.

I've had similar dreams to the one from which I was just awakened. Oh, to be able to play the guitar again or to pick up that paintbrush and finish the landscape art for my Mom. But, now, my hands are just gnarled flesh.

Leprosy is an extraordinary struggle but more so mentally than physically. There is therapy for my hands and effective medicine for this disease, but there's the deeper wound...the damage to your "will to live" from the infection of being forgotten."

The dream ended.

> *Remember, a small light will do a great deal when it is in a very dark place. -- DWIGHT L. MOODY*

For some inexplicable reason, I assumed lepers had been lepers all their lives. Wrapped in that assumption was an even more inexplicable thought—because they had not experienced normalcy nor experienced a regular life, they were spared the trauma of knowing what is missing and that somehow not having such common experiences lessens their agony. More to the shameful point, it allowed me to lessen my empathy for them, which lessened the guilt for me.

How tragically wrong I was.

As my brief dream illustrated for me, these were ordinary people, busily going about what any one of us would consider usual activities, when this disease unexpectedly interjected itself into their lives. Since then, little has been normal, regular, or ordinary about their lives. Faced with a similar challenge, who among us wouldn't be haunted by the memories of those times when our life was enjoyable, with a welcomed small measure of mundane?

What did I do to deserve being born in a prosperous country and not a developing country? What did I do to have the complete use of my physical abilities and not face the challenges of leprosy? What did I do to have the privileges, freedoms, and opportunities to enjoy and not suffer from an oppressive government, a malnourished health system, and a regressive educational structure?

The light shines in the darkness; and the darkness can never extinguish it. John 1:5 (NIV)

CHAPTER 13

MY PLEA (TO GOD)

Go away from me, Lord; I am a sinful man! Luke 5:8 (NIV)

WHAT DIFFERENCE will it make in this world if a leper in this faraway land is reached for You?

Why take the time to share the Gospel in such a backward place surrounded by the false teachings of other religions?

How can my presence, my words, adequately describe Your goodness, touch hearts in a healing way, and overcome generations of spiritual darkness?

Would it do any good to pour out my weaknesses to You? Surely our hearts cannot be divided about where these lepers belong in Your sky? I do not want them to live without You, but I cannot catch each of their tears. From the depths of my soul, I want all of them to live within Your promises. It is not enough that they suffered so much on this earth, that they must watch Your love fade from a distance because of me? Does their road to understanding have to go through me?

Don't show me what to do, just do it. Why should their eternity rely on my efforts? Just this once, please take this responsibility from me. I don't have enough courage, patience, or understanding to draw them from the shadows of this life to Your side.

They are barely holding on; it is uncertain how much longer they can wait on me. You hold time in Your hands. Would it be possible to not let time go through Your fingers quite as fast for a while? They deserve a better life. They deserve a better Christian—a Christian who can break their chains of anguish and set them free to roam Your fields of grace.

Why have you broken my heart for these people? There are too many pieces for me to pick up myself. Tell me there is a plan beyond just me. I am calling out to You to show them the world as You see it. It is asking too much for me to bring unnumbered others' heartbeats in line with Yours.

I don't want to feel this way anymore. This ache is everywhere I go. There is nothing remaining to do than surrender my place to one of them. I must let You go. Maybe that is where my life will begin again? Do I dare?

It is better than disappointing You. These people are worth more than my entering Your kingdom. I am begging You to open wide the gates to Your eternal love to them and allow Your goodness to bless them in ways they could never imagine. I know You see them. Please don't let their tears fall from my face.

I am hoping, this once, You will intervene. I am a simple, fallen man crying out from my corrupted soul to not let these lepers and their families fade away from Your heart. The promise of a glorious future cannot always make sense to the present sufferer. It is Your voice, not mine, they need to hear.

How can You allow those with so little to leave with even less?

Let not those who hope in you be ashamed because of me.
Psalm 69:6 (NIV)

61

CHAPTER 14

MY PLEA (TO YOU)

You do not know what tomorrow will bring. What is your life? For you are a mist that appears for a little time and then disappears. James 4:14 (NIV)

If we value our relationship with God, shouldn't we have in us the unconditional desire to help these people? If Jesus Christ is in us, shouldn't we defer to His way?

Our inactions suggest to those on the outside that our Christianity is hollow and selfish. As a result, there is no peace for us or hope for them.

So many of us are dishonoring our love for God because we have grown content with our own blessings and are unwilling to even temporarily suffer so others may experience His love. Isn't it our responsibility to love one another regardless of color, culture, or character?

As others are tossed between hope and fear, isn't it our responsibility, as Christians, to be trusted sources of spiritual refreshment—to help strengthen their resolve for the challenges they are facing?

Are you willing to help turn their hearts toward God for their eternal hope; to heal their contorted souls by encouraging them to look to Him for inner peace; to deliver them from their fears of loneliness, isolation, and desperation by sharing the love and friendship that awaits them by believing in Jesus Christ?

Who Better Than You?

It seems clear that, for too many of us, there are places we will not go and people we will not serve. For His glory, exercise the courage to ask God to change your heart.

Go beyond the ordinary, go beyond your reasoning, and use your talents, before God gives the privilege to sacrifice for another to someone else. Don't deny God the opportunity to work through you, to share His unconditional love and timeless truth with the suffering lepers of Myanmar.

We need to move past the fascination with the disease of leprosy and the novelty of seeing a leper. This isn't about using hurting people as an antidote for curing our spiritual wounds. It is about proving our worthiness to be faithful servants when life is at its height of uncertainty. Lepers have relevance to our spiritual lives—petitioning our hearts to care for strangers in a distant land, to provide us with a glimpse into our souls to see more fully who God intended us to be—a wonderful work, a triumph of creation, a servant who loves without bounds.

It is time for spiritual honesty, a time for the Christian community to hold itself accountable to the highest moral standards it professes. The purpose of our visits to such places as a leprosy hospital is not about scoring spiritual points, but to refine ourselves while helping the spiritually lost to better understand their suffering in the light of our God's love and truth. Such an achievement is not beyond our ability when we place ourselves in the purposeful hands of God.

We know what we should do. Someday we will be asked about our response to His appeal to our hearts, so demand from yourself the faith to yield your next step to the God through whom all things are possible.

Myanmar is God's land. We shouldn't underestimate what God is already doing among the people of Myanmar. God has prepared minds and hearts in this hospital and village to receive, understand, and accept the words of hope we are personally responsible for sharing. For someone, your story is the only one they have been prepared to hear.

They are waiting, but on whom they don't know. Are you willing to help their hearts find a home?

Why Go?

Perhaps it is better for us to stay home, to retreat from the heartache we read about. What can we accomplish in a few weeks anyway? Why disturb our own peace to stir the ashes of hope among others? After all, each of us will be held accountable for our unbelief whether a scripture is shared, a Bible is given, or a sermon is delivered. The evidence of God is available to any seeking heart, without us punishing ourselves to be personally by their sides.

Surely, one of us has the patience to seduce their troubling outlook on life with the lure of God's unconditional love, on which a true foundation of inner peace can be built.

We all know they need more than just encouraging words. We all know the right thing to do. We need to point their hearts to the Lord. It isn't enough to pray they will be all right. We need to help them find their way. Their hearts are willing to take the chance, their souls are willing to live, but their hope is far beneath their courage, and all they can see are their struggles.

They keep fighting an internal battle against that voice whispering they are unworthy. We must help them see where to go, understand what they are missing, and realize hope is within their reach. They need to hear God speak, to tell them they are loved, to tell them they are not forgotten, to tell them who they really are—His!

What are we afraid of? Are we concerned about what they will think when we share about Christianity? Of course, it will take more than our words, it will take the Holy Spirit to help them unravel the love story of Christianity. Although we can't save anyone, we can't leave our life-changing stories behind, like treasures without a map, to be hopefully stumbled on.

There are few feelings better than the one believing God has used you to serve others successfully. The joy inside your soul is immeasurable when you fulfill His purpose, in whatever circumstances He has placed you. Whether it is on an African plain, a vacant lot in an American ghetto, or a leprosy hospital in Myanmar, the focus should not be on the work itself but rather your relationship with God.

It is important that we not weigh down our decision about whether "to go" with an analysis of our usefulness. We should be unbound by any thoughts of God having starved us of gifts to use for serving others. Don't swerve around God's calling, thinking somehow you are inadequate.

The reality is all we must do is follow where He leads, bringing all our fears and frailties, because the results are not dependent on our efforts but His. Let's not revel in our perceived shortcomings but honor God through a faith that focuses on His glory, not ours.

Keep in mind that "our going" may not be so we can be the answer or source of comfort for someone but be a fellow sufferer. We shouldn't consider that God's plan for us is always to be the glimmer of Christianity for someone. At times, we should be prepared to be the one for whom others will be the light, for whom others will be blessed by shining their kindness and understanding on us.

By "not going," we risk being an incomplete design either by not experiencing a personal blessing by serving another or being a blessing for another. We must be willing to suffer, to be placed in trying circumstances, to be surrounded by discouragement.

Don't go through your life wondering what God could have done through you. Be the answer to your own prayer about helping these lepers and their families.

Why Now?

You may be thinking that interacting with lepers is well beyond your capabilities. You may have already thought of an array of excuses to convince yourself you are the wrong person. However, this is one of those rare God-given opportunities when the cost to ourselves is certain but helping others "find their way" is the purpose of a lifetime. This is an opportunity to do something beyond yourself, to become the person God designed by becoming the difference in someone else's life.

The battlefield is not on the Leprosy Hospital grounds. It is in the chambers of our hearts where the fears of the moment go to great lengths to expose our fragile beliefs and values.

Use your faith to show them the hope in your religion is a promise, a blessing which reaches those unknown places in your life, healing and nourishing your soul.

I know you do not want to deprive these lepers and their families from knowing your God. I know you do not want them to continue in their lives believing they deserve to be rejected by this world. I know you have the courage, no matter the personal cost, to go where you have never been. I know you feel spiritually fragile and unsure even what to pray, but admitting your doubts allows you the pleasure of feeling God's presence, as well as his protection.

Carefully camouflaged motives centered on personal achievements rather than kingdom building can lead to bad choices and major spiritual damage. We can deceive ourselves into believing we are acting honorably; after all, lepers are "the least of these," and helping them goes against the vast majority's natural sense of brotherly love. It is one thing to "go," but to love someone that is different from you reduces the servants to a handful. It is about loving strangers.

There is a risk to reaching out, connecting, loving others. There is a responsibility to surrendering our comfort, our time, our blessings for others. There is a reward to giving your heart, sharing your story, and overcoming your fears for others.

What can well-meaning people do at this place? Is it possible to make a difference when stepping into a world with few choices? Is it enough to pray and trust God with their care? Some of us never consider doing anything more. What a tragedy! From whom will these lepers learn about Jesus Christ?

Don't spend too many days wondering. It is your decision to either share the "Good News" or keep the "Good News" from them. You can push your questions only slightly out of sight, but eventually you must think about them: Is it necessary to travel 10,000 miles to share your faith? Wouldn't your energies be better invested sharing the Gospel with people who have no religion at all than trying to convince persons with entrenched beliefs? If you feel compelled "to go," shouldn't you consider a place where the odds are more favorable?

Do you know yourself well enough to tell yourself the truth? Once you do, you will have the foundation on which to share the Gospel honestly with others. The timing and the details to ensure a meaningful experience is in God's hands.

Fast-forward, imagine someone is listening to stories of how these lepers and their family members came to know the Lord. Imagine the inspiration they have been to others.

Imagine hearing how they had not only encouraged one another but led others to Christ. Imagine the remarkable privilege to know that it all started when you took that first step of faith to travel to Myanmar.

Together, let's shake the heavens!

This generation of Christians is responsible for this generation of souls on the earth. -- KEITH GREEN, Christian Composer and Musician

CHAPTER 15

WHEN (A PRAYER FOR YOU)

Do not fritter away your life in thinking of what you intend to do tomorrow. No man ever served God by doing things tomorrow. -- CHARLES SPURGEON

MY PARTING WORDS are from bended knees. As Christians, we have the privilege in our troubled times to share our sorrows with our Lord. However, our souls are in constant danger from the worldly desires we find so difficult to leave behind. Despite our bests efforts to surrender our lives completely to Him, at times, love is not so easy to see in this world, in ourselves, or express to others.

Nonetheless, we cannot be distracted by the charms of this world. God sees us. God hears us. He knows how each of us ended up here. He remains in control. It is my prayer that His love surrounds your soul, protects your hopes, and brings your heart out from hiding because there are hurting people on the other side of the world—waiting.

In those times when you start to turn your back on what you know you should do, may you rediscover God's plan for you.

In those times when you are disillusioned with Christianity's promises, may you reconnect to its divine strategy and moral principles.

In those times when your poor choices lead to suffering, may you value repentance and turn back toward God.

In those times when you are justifying your self-interests, may you realize you have been given the inner strength to suppress their appeal.

In those times when you harshly judge others, may you come to understand your views are not harmless speculations.

In those times when your expectations are replaced with sorrow, may you find peace in knowing God is working to carry out what is in your best interests.

In those times when you think your way is best, may you get redirected by faith to trust what you cannot see.

In those times when you feel harmed, may you find freedom from your pain in the joy of forgiveness.

In those times when you struggle to understand God, may you find reassurance of His goodness through serving others.

In those times when you are looking for relevance in your life, may you be in that place where God invited you to serve— in that one place where His eyes will be looking just for you.

One never leaves Myanmar as they entered!

JOIN US

WE WELCOME YOUR PARTICIPATION on one of our annual mission trips to Myanmar, to visit the Leprosy Hospital personally. Should you be interested in joining us on a trip, wish to contribute to our leprosy ministry, or learn more about our organization, you can reach us at:

Love for Myanmar
305 Ten Oaks Drive
Georgetown, Texas 78633
www.loveformyanmar.org
(512) 562-2455

Examples of Needs

The following items are provided as examples of the needs of the hospital. It is not a comprehensive list or provided in any order of priority.

These items are legitimate needs, from among many, and chosen to provide prospective donors with an idea of how their financial gifts will be used. Because conditions can change, priorities can change, and it is therefore preferred that your contributions be given without designating a specific item.

The LFM staff is continually in communication with the staff of the Leprosy Hospital. We assure you that 100% of your contributions will be provided to the Leprosy Hospital ministry, based on whatever priorities are currently identified by the Leprosy Hospital staff:

- Crutches, walkers, and wheelchairs
- Adjustable operating beds
- Oxygen bottles
- Anesthesia machine with IV line
- Patient monitors
- Facilities Improvements: Incinerator for medical waste
- Painting of wards
- Transformer (50 KVA) Generator (10 KVA)
- Refurbishing staff houses on the compound
- Training:
- Physiotherapy (restoring function and motion)
- Occupational Therapy (helping children with disabilities)
- Orthopedic Technology (casting, splinting of bones and joints)

You can make your tax-deductible donation by check payable to *Love for Myanmar,* with a designation to the Leprosy Ministry, and mail it to:

Love for Myanmar
305 Ten Oaks Drive
Georgetown, Texas 78633

If you prefer, you can donate online by visiting our website:
www.loveformyanmar.org

Resources

As you consider becoming involved in our leprosy ministry, you are encouraged to read, *The Gift of Pain*, by Dr. Paul Brand and Philip Yancey. Dr. Brand is a leprosy specialist, and Mr. Yancey is an award-winning author. Their collaboration unwraps the unique world in which lepers live.

Other recommended resources on leprosy:

- American Leprosy Missions https://www.leprosy.org/
- Infolep: international knowledge center on leprosy https://www.leprosy-information.org/
- International Federation of Anti-Leprosy Associations http://www.ilepfederation.org/

ABOUT THE AUTHOR

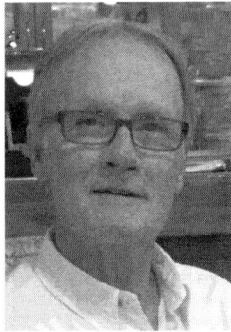

My blessings are too numerous to include here; however, the following are among those to highlight for their relevance to this book.

I was raised by Christian parents with an understanding that people matter and deserve your kindness and respect; and was blessed with the continual mentoring you should care about how you live your faith.

I earned degrees in political science and public administration and was blessed with the opportunity to be employed for decades within an organization which truly strived to make our public a better place.

I am blessed to be married nearly 50 years to the only person whom God entrusted with the monumental task of understanding my thinking, and the willingness to endure its periodic mystery while sharing the joys of two wonderful sons.

I am blessed to be involved in a church which appreciates the value of missions and invests its resources to facilitate the involvement of its members and others in the Great Commission throughout its region, its State, its country, and in some of the spiritually darkest places on our earth.

Printed in Great Britain
by Amazon